THE 5 MINUTE PAIN-FREE KNEE ARTHRITIS EXERCISE

FOR SENIORS OVER 50

Easy Workout Plan Ranging From Yoga, Stretching, Chair Props & Tai Chi to Heal Kneel & Joint Pains, prevent falls and boost balance.

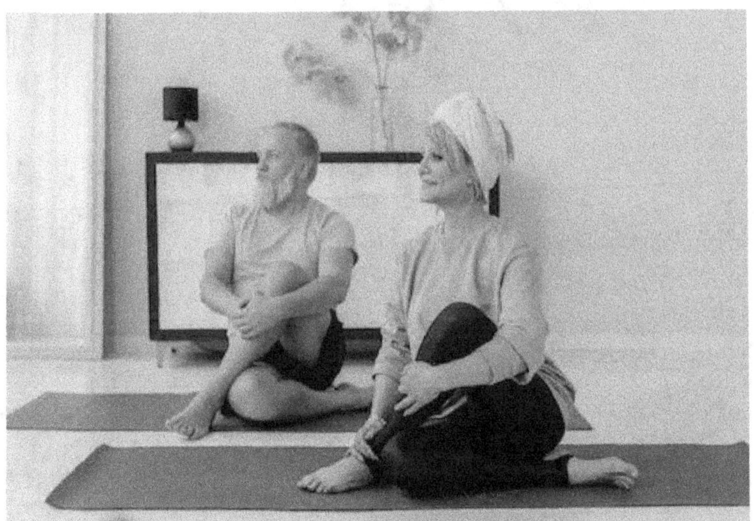

DR. KADEN WINTON

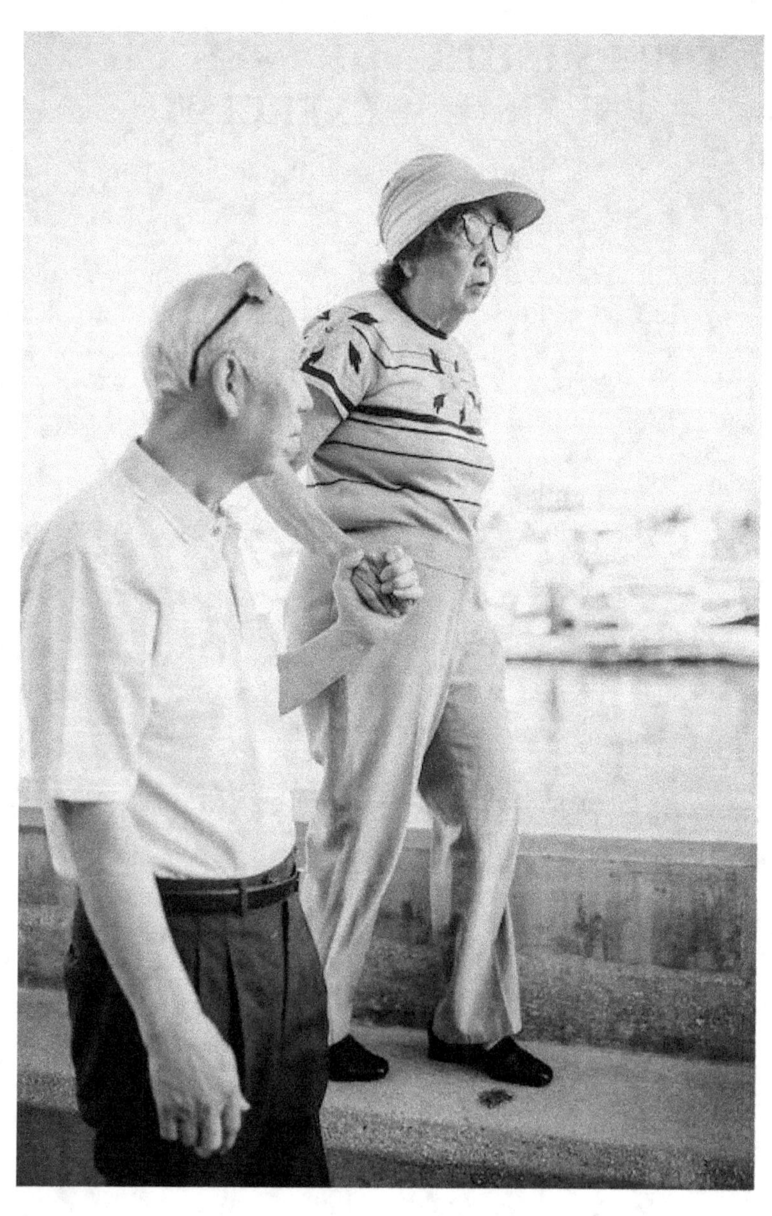

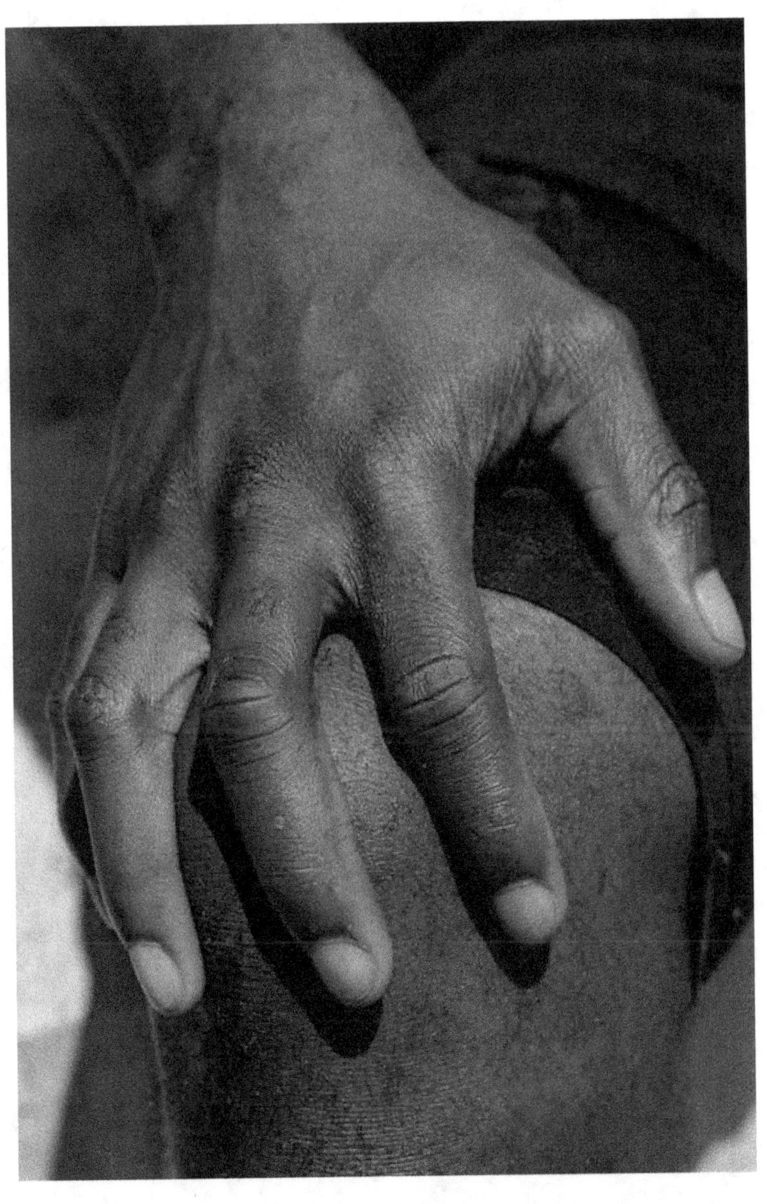

Table of Contents

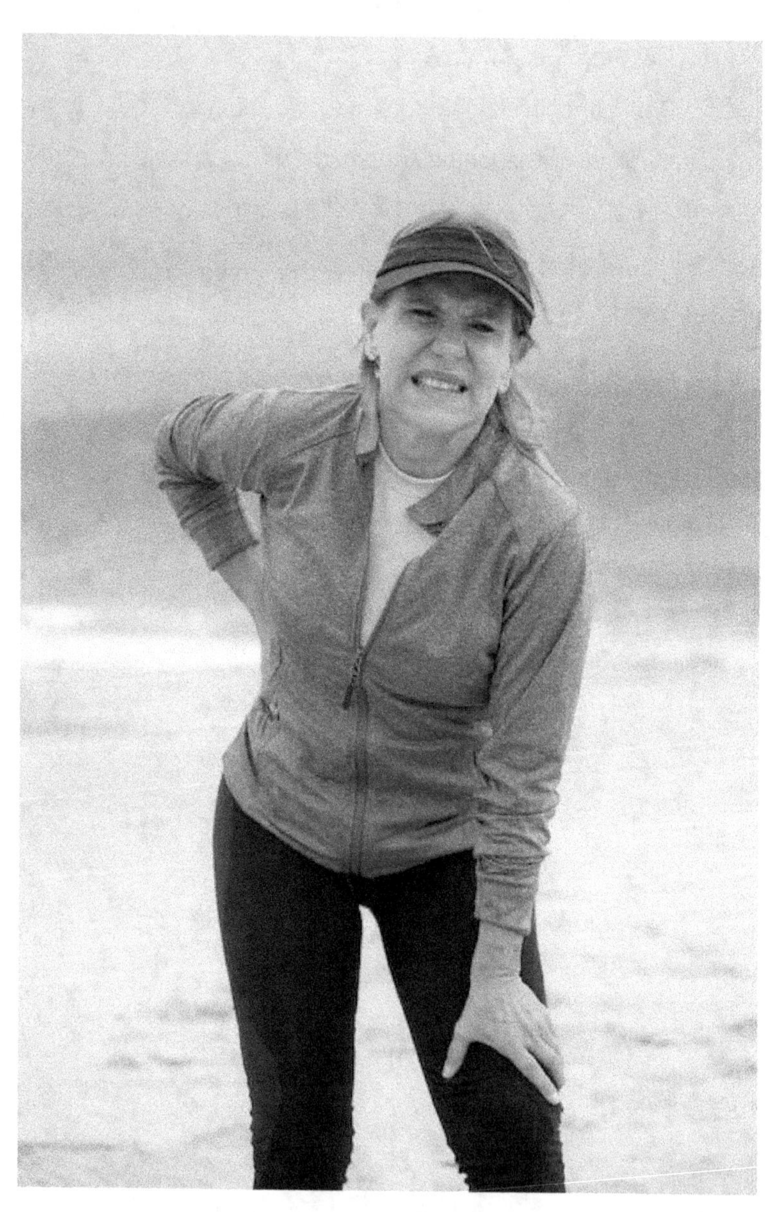

Introduction

John had always been an active and independent senior. At 65, he had enjoyed a life filled with outdoor adventures and sports. But lately, something had been slowing him down. He started experiencing nagging discomfort and stiffness in his knees, making it difficult to keep up with his beloved activities. However, being the resilient man, John brushed off the symptoms, assuming they were just signs of aging.

As time went by, the pain in his knees became unbearable. Walking even short distances became a struggle, and climbing stairs became daunting. Finally, John couldn't ignore it any longer. He made an appointment with his doctor and underwent a series of tests. The results were not surprising - John was diagnosed with knee arthritis.

The doctor prescribed medications to alleviate the pain and suggested physical therapy. Though grateful for the diagnosis and treatment plan, John still longed for a solution to bring him back to a pain-free life. He had no idea how his life would soon change.

One evening, while browsing the internet for any information that could help him find relief, John stumbled upon a post by Dr. Kaden Winton. The post discussed pain-free knee exercises specifically designed for seniors with arthritis. Intrigued, John read every word, soaking in the information.

Motivated by newfound hope, John decided to give the exercises a try. He dedicated five minutes each day to performing the gentle movements and stretches outlined by Dr. Winton. Gradually, he started noticing a difference. The pain began to diminish, and his mobility improved.

Weeks turned into months, and John's perseverance paid off. The exercises became an integral part of his daily routine. Not only did he regain his mobility, but he also discovered a renewed sense of vitality. He could walk without discomfort, climb stairs effortlessly, and engage in activities he thought were forever lost to him.

Filled with gratitude, John couldn't thank Dr. Kaden Winton enough for sharing his expertise. He knew that his life had been forever changed by the simple yet powerful exercises that freed him from knee arthritis.

Inspired by his journey, John shared his experience with others, hoping to offer them the same transformative solution he had found. With a newfound purpose, he embarked on a mission to spread awareness about the life-changing potential of pain-free knee exercises for seniors over 50.

Knee arthritis is a condition that affects millions of people worldwide, particularly seniors over the age of 50. It can significantly impact one's quality of life, limiting mobility and causing chronic pain. Understanding knee arthritis is crucial to manage and treat this condition effectively. This article will delve into the various aspects of knee arthritis, including its definition, causes, risk factors, symptoms, diagnosis, and treatment options.

What is Knee Arthritis?

Knee arthritis, also known as osteoarthritis of the knee, is a degenerative joint disease characterized by the gradual wearing down of the cartilage in the knee joint. The knee joint is composed of the femur (thighbone), tibia (shinbone), and patella (kneecap). The smooth cartilage lining these bones helps facilitate smooth movement. In knee arthritis, this cartilage gradually deteriorates, leading to pain, stiffness, and reduced mobility.

Causes and Risk Factors

Knee arthritis can develop as a result of numerous factors. Age is a significant factor, as the wear and tear on the knee joint increase over time. Other causes include obesity, previous knee injuries or surgeries, genetic predisposition, and repetitive stress on the knee joint.

Symptoms and Diagnosis

From person to person, knee arthritis symptoms can differ. Common signs include pain, stiffness, swelling, decreased range of motion, and a grating sensation during movement.

Diagnosis typically involves a comprehensive evaluation by a healthcare professional, including a physical examination, medical history review, and imaging tests such as X-rays and MRI scans.

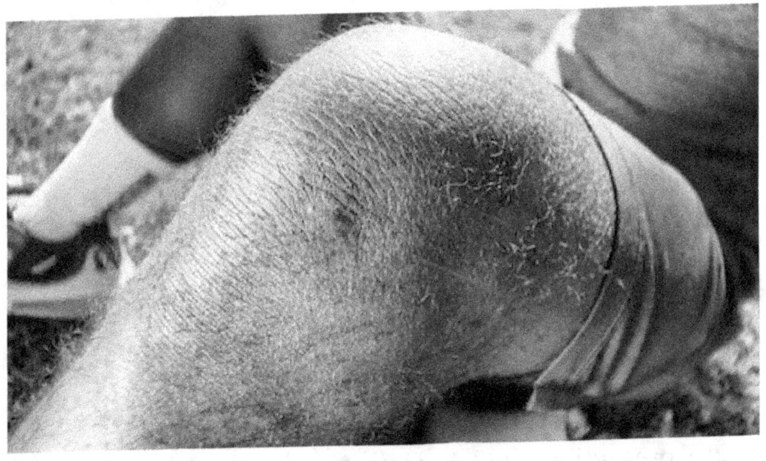

In the following chapters of this book, we will be evaluating the connection between arthritis an exercise a well as quick and easy exercises to promote arthritis healing.

Chapter One

Exercise and Knee Arthritis

Knee arthritis can be debilitating, causing pain, stiffness, and reduced mobility. However, exercise has emerged as a vital component in managing and treating knee arthritis. Contrary to common misconceptions, appropriate and regular physical activity can alleviate pain, improve joint function, and enhance overall well-being. In this comprehensive article, we will delve into the importance of exercise for knee arthritis, explore its numerous benefits, and provide essential safety precautions and guidelines for creating a safe and effective exercise routine.

Importance of Exercise for Knee Arthritis

Exercise is crucial for individuals with knee arthritis as it offers a range of benefits that can significantly improve their condition and overall quality of life. Firstly, regular exercise helps maintain joint flexibility and range of motion. Engaging in gentle, controlled movements helps lubricate the joints and reduce stiffness, enabling individuals to perform daily activities more easily.

Moreover, exercise plays a pivotal role in strengthening the muscles surrounding the knee joint. Strong muscles provide better support and stability, reducing the strain on the knee and alleviating pain. Individuals can enhance joint function and reduce the risk of further injury by improving muscular strength and endurance.

Additionally, exercise promotes weight management, which is particularly important for individuals with knee arthritis. Overweight people put more strain on their knee joints, which makes them more painful and hastens joint aging. By incorporating exercise into a comprehensive weight management plan, individuals can reduce the burden on their knees, enhancing their overall well-being and mobility.

Furthermore, exercise has positive effects on mental health. Endorphins, which naturally elevate mood, are secreted when you exercise. Regular exercise can reduce stress, anxiety, and depression, improving overall psychological well-being.

Regular exercise offers many benefits for individuals with knee arthritis, encompassing physical and mental well-being. Let's delve deeper into a few of these advantages:

a. Improved Joint Function and Mobility

Regular exercise helps improve joint flexibility and range of motion, making it easier to perform daily activities such as walking, climbing stairs, and bending. Engaging in exercises that target the lower body, such as leg stretches and range-of-motion exercises, can enhance joint mobility and reduce stiffness.

b. Strengthened Muscles and Joint Support

Exercise plays a vital role in strengthening the muscles surrounding the knee joint. Stronger muscles provide better support and stability, reducing the stress on the knee and decreasing pain. Exercises such as leg raises, squats and lunges can target the quadriceps, hamstrings, and glutes, helping to alleviate knee discomfort.

c. Weight Management and Reduced Strain on Joints

Excess weight significantly strains the knee joints, exacerbating pain and accelerating joint degeneration. Regular exercise and a healthy diet can contribute to weight loss or maintenance, reducing the burden on the knees and improving joint health.

d. Improved Cardiovascular Health

Cardiovascular exercises such as walking, cycling, swimming, or water aerobics can improve heart health and overall fitness. These low-impact activities provide a cardiovascular workout while minimizing stress on the knees.

e. Reduced Inflammation and Pain

Exercise helps reduce inflammation in the body, including the knee joints. Low-impact exercises can stimulate the production of synovial fluid, a natural lubricant that nourishes the joints and reduces pain. Regular physical activity also triggers the release of endorphins, natural pain-relieving chemicals that can help alleviate discomfort.

f. Enhanced Balance and Stability

Certain exercises like balance and stability can help improve proprioception and coordination. These exercises focus on strengthening the muscles responsible for balance and stability, reducing the risk of falls and injuries.

g. Improved Mental Well-being

Exercise has significant mental health benefits, promoting positive mood and reducing stress, anxiety, and depression. Engaging in physical activity can serve as a form of therapy, providing a sense of accomplishment and improving overall psychological well-being.

Safety Precautions and Guidelines

While exercise benefits individuals with knee arthritis, it is essential to approach it cautiously to prevent exacerbating pain or causing further injury. Here are some important safety precautions and guidelines to consider:

a. Consult with a Healthcare Professional

Before starting any exercise routine, it is crucial to consult with your healthcare provider or a physical therapist. They can evaluate your condition, provide personalized recommendations, and help design an exercise program tailored to your needs and limitations.

b. Choose Low-Impact Exercises

Opt for low-impact exercises that reduce knee stress while still providing cardiovascular benefits. Activities such as walking, cycling, swimming, water aerobics, or using an elliptical machine are excellent options. These exercises promote joint mobility and cardiovascular fitness without placing excessive knee strain.

c. Warm-up and Cool-down

Always start your exercise session with a proper warm-up to prepare the muscles and joints for activity. This can include light aerobic exercises and gentle stretches. Similarly, end the session with a cool-down period involving light stretching exercises and gradual slowing of activity. Warm-up and cool-down routines are crucial for injury prevention and reducing muscle soreness.

d. Gradual Progression

Start with gentle exercises and gradually increase the duration and intensity over time. Listening to your body and avoiding pushing yourself too hard is essential, as it can lead to overexertion and increased pain. The risk of injury is reduced by gradual progression, which enables your body to adjust to the demands of exercise.

e. Focus on Proper Form and Technique

Maintaining proper form and technique during exercises is essential for minimizing knee strain and maximizing benefits. Work with a physical therapist to ensure correct posture, alignment, and movement patterns if needed.

f. Modify or Avoid High-Impact Activities

High-impact activities like running or jumping can place excessive stress on the knee joints. If you enjoy such activities, consider alternative low-impact options like using an elliptical machine or stationary cycling. Modifying exercises or utilizing equipment such as knee braces can help protect the joints during physical activity.

Chapter Two

Getting Started

Regular exercise is crucial for managing knee arthritis and improving joint mobility. The 5-minute exercise routine offers a convenient and time-efficient way for seniors over 50 to incorporate physical activity into their daily lives. This extensive article will guide you through getting started with the 5-minute exercise routine. We will explore the importance of preparing for exercise, the significance of warm-up and stretching, and the essential equipment needed to maximize the effectiveness and safety of your workout.

Preparing for Exercise

Before embarking on any exercise routine, preparing your body and mind for physical activity is essential. Here are some crucial steps to take into account:

a. Consult with a Healthcare Professional

If you have any pre-existing medical conditions or concerns, it is crucial to consult with your healthcare provider before starting the 5-minute exercise routine. They can provide personalized guidance, taking into account your specific needs and limitations.

b. Set Realistic Goals

Establish clear and realistic goals for your exercise routine. These goals include increasing joint flexibility, reducing pain, or improving overall fitness. By setting achievable goals, you can stay motivated and track your progress.

c. Create a Schedule

Incorporate the 5-minute exercise routine into your daily schedule. Consistency is crucial for getting the most benefit from exercise. Choose a specific time of day that works best for you and stick to it.

d. Find a Suitable Exercise Space

Identify a suitable exercise space in your home or outdoors where you can comfortably perform the routine. Ensure the area is well-lit, spacious, and free from obstacles to minimize the risk of accidents or injuries.

Chapter Three

The Comprehensive 5-Minute Pain-Free Knee Arthritis Exercise Routine

The 5-minute pain-free knee arthritis exercise routine consists of exercises targeting joint health, muscle strength, balance, and flexibility. This extensive guide will delve into each exercise in detail, providing step-by-step instructions to ensure proper form and maximum benefit. By incorporating these exercises into your daily routine, you can effectively manage knee arthritis, improve joint mobility, strengthen supporting muscles, enhance balance and stability, and alleviate pain and discomfort.

Low-Impact 5-Minute Aerobic Exercises for Arthritis

Low-impact aerobic exercises are an excellent choice for individuals with arthritis as they provide cardiovascular benefits without placing excessive stress on the joints. This comprehensive guide will explore three low-impact aerobic exercises designed to help individuals with arthritis maintain a healthy cardiovascular system, improve endurance, and support joint health. These exercises can be easily incorporated into a 5-minute routine and offer numerous benefits for overall well-being.

Exercise 1: Walking

Walking is a simple yet highly effective low-impact aerobic exercise that individuals of all fitness levels can perform. Here's how to maximize the benefits of walking for arthritis:

- Start with a gentle warm-up by walking comfortably for a few minutes.
- Gradually increase your pace to a brisk walk, maintaining good posture and swinging your arms naturally.
- Aim to walk for 5 minutes at a steady and consistent pace, focusing on engaging the muscles of your legs and core.
- Pay attention to your body's signals and adjust the intensity or duration if needed.
- To add variety to your routine, consider walking on different surfaces such as grass, gravel, or sand, as this can engage different muscles and challenge your balance.

Exercise 2: Cycling

Cycling is a low-impact aerobic exercise that provides cardiovascular benefits while minimizing joint stress. Follow these steps to perform a 5-minute cycling exercise for arthritis:

- If using a stationary bike, adjust the seat height to ensure proper alignment of your knees and hips.
- Begin with a gentle warm-up, pedaling comfortably for a few minutes.
- Gradually increase the resistance or speed to a moderate intensity that challenges you but does not cause pain or discomfort.
- Maintain this intensity for 5 minutes, focusing on maintaining good posture and engaging the muscles of your legs and core.
- If you prefer outdoor cycling, choose flat terrain or use a stationary bike with adjustable resistance to simulate outdoor cycling.

Exercise 3: Water Aerobics

Water aerobics is a low-impact exercise that provides resistance and support, making it ideal for individuals with arthritis. Here's how to perform a 5-minute water aerobics routine:

- Find a pool with water that is chest-deep or at a comfortable height for your abilities.
- Begin with a gentle warm-up by walking or marching in place, lifting your knees, and swinging your arms.
- Progress to different exercises such as leg kicks, arm movements, and torso twists, all performed in the water.
- Aim to perform a variety of movements for 5 minutes, focusing on maintaining proper form and engaging the muscles of your body.
- The water's buoyancy reduces the impact on your joints while providing resistance, helping to strengthen your muscles and improve cardiovascular fitness.

Incorporating low-impact aerobic exercises into your daily routine can significantly benefit individuals with arthritis. Walking, cycling, and water aerobics are excellent choices for maintaining cardiovascular health and supporting joint function. Following the step-by-step instructions for each exercise, you can create a 5-minute routine that promotes endurance, strengthens muscles, and improves overall well-being. Always start slowly, pay attention to your body, and gradually increase the duration and intensity of your workouts. Consistency and dedication to these low-impact aerobic exercises will help you manage arthritis symptoms, enhance joint health, and lead a healthier, more active lifestyle.

Five-Minute Range of Motion Exercises for Knee Arthritis: Enhancing Joint Flexibility and Reducing Stiffness

Range of motion exercises are crucial in managing knee arthritis by improving joint flexibility, reducing stiffness, and enhancing overall mobility. In this comprehensive guide, we will explore some five-minute range of motion exercises specifically designed to target the knees and alleviate the symptoms of knee arthritis. These exercises can be easily incorporated into your daily routine and offer numerous benefits for maintaining joint health and functionality.

Exercise 4: Knee Flexion and Extension

Knee flexion and extension exercises are fundamental for increasing the range of motion in the knees and promoting flexibility. Follow these tailored steps to perform this exercise:

- Sit on a chair with your back straight and feet flat on the floor.
- Slowly lift one leg off the ground and extend it before you.
- Gradually flex your knee, bringing your foot back towards your buttocks.
- Hold the flexed position for a few seconds, feeling a gentle stretch in the front of your thigh.
- Slowly extend your leg back out before you, straightening your knee.
- Repeat this movement 10 times for each leg, focusing on controlled and smooth motions.

- Gradually increase the range of motion as tolerated, but avoid any movements that cause pain or discomfort.

Exercise 5: Knee Circles

Knee circles are effective for promoting joint mobility and reducing knee stiffness. Here's how to perform knee circles:

- Sit on a chair with your back straight and feet flat on the floor.
- Lift one leg off the ground and bend your knee, bringing your foot towards your buttocks.
- Slowly rotate your knee in a circular motion, clockwise or counterclockwise.
- Focus on making the circles as large as possible while maintaining comfort and control.
- Perform 5 circles in one direction and then switch to the opposite direction.
- Repeat the exercise with the other leg, aiming for 10 circles in each direction.

Exercise 6: Heel Slides

Heel slides effectively improve knee flexion and increase the range of motion in the knees. Follow these steps to perform heel slides:

- Lie on your back on a flat surface with your legs extended.
- Slowly slide one heel towards your buttocks, bending your knee as much as possible.
- For a few seconds, maintain the bent position while feeling a light stretch in the front of your thigh.
- Slowly slide your heel back out, straightening your knee.
- Repeat this movement 10 times for each leg, focusing on controlled and smooth motions.
- Gradually increase the range of motion as tolerated, but stop if you experience pain or discomfort.

Exercise 7: Straight Leg Raises

Straight leg raises effectively strengthen the quadriceps muscles and improve knee stability. Here's how to perform this exercise:

- Sit on a chair with your back straight and feet flat on the floor.

- Straighten one leg before you, keeping your knee straight.

- Slowly lift your leg off the ground, aiming to bring it parallel to the floor.

- Maintain the raised position while contracting your quadriceps for a few seconds.

- Slowly lower your leg back down.

- Repeat this movement 10 times for each leg, focusing on controlled and smooth motions.

Exercise 8: Ankle Pumps

Ankle pumps help improve circulation and flexibility in the ankles, indirectly benefiting the knees. Follow these tailored steps to perform ankle pumps:

- Sit on a chair with your back straight and feet flat on the floor.

- Lift both feet off the ground, keeping your knees bent.

- Point your toes downward, feeling a stretch in the front of your ankles.

- Slowly flex your feet upward, pointing your toes towards the ceiling.

- Repeat this pumping motion 10 times, aiming for a smooth and continuous movement.

Incorporating a range of motion exercises into your daily routine is essential for managing knee arthritis. The exercises evaluated above - knee flexion and extension, knee circles, heel slides, straight leg raises, and ankle pumps - are effective for improving joint flexibility, reducing stiffness, and increasing the range of motion in the knees. Following the step-by-step instructions for each exercise, you can create a five-minute routine that targets the knees and promotes better joint health. Remember to start slowly, listen to your body, and adjust the exercises to your comfort and ability level. Consistency and dedication to these range of motion exercises will help alleviate the symptoms of knee arthritis, enhance joint mobility, and improve your overall quality of life.

Five Minutes Strengthening Exercises for Knee Arthritis: Building Stability and Support

Strengthening exercises are vital for individuals with knee arthritis as they help build stability, improve muscle strength, and support the knees. In this comprehensive guide, we will explore essential strengthening exercises specifically designed to target the muscles around the knees, alleviate pain, and enhance overall joint function. These exercises can be easily incorporated into your daily routine and offer numerous benefits for maintaining strong and healthy knees.

Exercise 9: Quadriceps Sets

Quadriceps sets effectively strengthen the quadriceps muscles, which play a crucial role in knee stability. Follow these steps to perform quadriceps sets:

- Sit on a chair with your back straight and feet flat on the floor.
- Straighten one leg before you, keeping your knee straight.
- Tighten the muscles on the front of your thigh (quadriceps) and hold the contraction for 5-10 seconds.

- Release the contraction and relax your leg.

- Repeat this exercise 10 times for each leg, focusing on controlled contractions and releases.

Exercise 10: Hamstring Curls

Hamstring curls target the muscles at the back of the thigh and help balance the strength between the front and back of the knee. Here's how to perform hamstring curls:

- Stand behind a chair, holding onto it for support.

- Bend one knee and bring your heel toward your buttocks, feeling a contraction in the back of your thigh (hamstring).

- Hold the curled position for a few seconds, then slowly lower your foot.

- Repeat this movement 10 times for each leg, focusing on controlled and smooth motions.

Exercise 11: Glute Bridges

Glute bridges engage the gluteal muscles and help improve hip and pelvic stability, indirectly supporting the knees. Follow these tailored steps to perform glute bridges:

- Lie on a flat surface with your knees bent and feet flat on the floor, hip-width apart.
- Press your heels into the floor and lift your buttocks off the ground, forming a straight line from your knees to your shoulders.
- Squeeze your gluteal muscles at the top of the bridge position, holding for a few seconds.
- Slowly lower your buttocks back down to the ground.
- Repeat this exercise 10 times, focusing on controlled and controlled movements.

Exercise 12: Wall Squats

Wall squats effectively strengthen the quadriceps, hamstrings, and gluteal muscles, providing stability and support to the knees. Here's how to perform wall squats:

- Your feet should be shoulder-width apart as you stand with your back against a wall.

- Slowly slide your back down the wall while bending your knees, as if sitting in an imaginary chair.

- Keep your knees aligned with your toes and go as far down as is comfortable.

- Hold this position for a few seconds, then push through your heels to return to standing.

- Repeat this exercise 10 times, focusing on controlled movements and maintaining proper form.

Exercise 13: Step-Ups

Step-ups target the quadriceps, hamstrings, and gluteal muscles while simulating movements involved in stair climbing. Follow these steps to perform step-ups:

- Find a sturdy step or platform that is around knee height.

- Step onto the platform with one foot, pushing through your heel and engaging your leg muscles.

- Lift your body onto the platform, straightening your knee.

- Step back down with the same foot, lowering yourself in a controlled manner.

- Repeat this exercise 10 times for each leg, alternating between legs.

Incorporating strengthening exercises into your daily routine is crucial for managing knee arthritis and promoting joint stability. The exercises mentioned above - quadriceps sets, hamstring curls, glute bridges, wall squats, and step-ups - target the key muscle groups around the knees, providing support and enhancing overall joint strength. Following the step-by-step instructions for each exercise, you can create a five-minute routine that focuses on strengthening the muscles around your knees. Remember to start slowly, listen to your body, and adjust the exercises to your comfort and ability level. Consistency and dedication to these strengthening exercises will help alleviate the symptoms of knee arthritis, improve muscle strength, and provide better support and stability to your knees.

Five Minutes Enhancing Balance and Stability Exercises for Knee Arthritis: Building Stability and Support

Maintaining balance and stability is crucial for individuals with knee arthritis, as it helps prevent falls, improves confidence in movement, and enhances overall quality of life. This comprehensive guide will explore five extensively effective balance and stability exercises specifically designed to target the muscles and systems responsible for maintaining equilibrium. These exercises can be easily incorporated into your daily routine and offer numerous benefits for improving balance and coordination and reducing the risk of falls.

Exercise 14: Single Leg Stance

The single-leg stance exercise is a foundational exercise that enhances balance and stability by engaging the muscles in the lower body. Follow these steps to perform the single-leg stance:

- Start by taking a tall stance and spreading your feet wide.
- Shift your weight onto one leg and lift the opposite foot slightly off the ground.
- To keep your posture upright, contract your core muscles.
- Find your balance and hold the position for 10-30 seconds.

- As you progress, challenge yourself by closing your eyes or performing small knee bends while maintaining balance.
- Repeat the exercise on the other leg, aiming for three sets on each side.

Exercise 15: Heel-to-Toe Walk

The heel-to-toe walk exercise is an excellent way to improve balance, coordination, and proprioception. Here's how to perform the heel-to-toe walk:

- Find a straight line on the ground, such as the edge of a carpet or a piece of tape.
- Begin by standing at one end of the line with relaxed arms.
- Place your right heel directly in front of your left toes, creating a heel-to-toe alignment.
- Take a step forward, bringing your left heel to touch the toes of your right foot.

- Continue this heel-to-toe pattern, walking along the line for 10-15 steps.

- Maintain a slow and deliberate pace, focusing on balance and alignment.

- If needed, you can have a stable object nearby for support.

Exercise 16: Standing Leg Swing

Standing leg swings are excellent exercises for improving balance, stability, and hip mobility. Follow these steps to perform standing leg swings:

- Put your hands on your hips while standing tall with your feet hip-width apart.

- Put all your weight on one leg while slightly bending your knee.

- Swing your opposite leg forward and backward in a controlled manner, maintaining balance throughout the movement.

- Aim for 10-15 swings on each leg, gradually increasing the height of the swing as you feel comfortable.

- To keep your balance and stability, contract your core muscles.

- If needed, you can hold onto a stable object for support.

Exercise 17: Tai Chi

Tai Chi is a traditional Chinese martial art emphasizing slow, flowing movements, deep breathing, and mindfulness. It has been widely recognized for its ability to improve balance, flexibility, and overall well-being. Consider joining a Tai Chi class or following instructional videos to learn and practice various Tai Chi movements that specifically target balance and stability.

Exercise 18: Yoga Tree Pose

The Tree poses in yoga are fantastic for enhancing balance, stability, and concentration. Follow these tailored steps to perform the Tree pose:

- Start by taking a tall stance, keeping your arms by your sides and your feet hip-width apart.
- Shift your weight onto one leg and bring the sole of your opposite foot to rest on the inner thigh of your standing leg.

- If you find it challenging to balance, you can place your foot on the calf or ankle instead.

- Find a focal point in front of you to help maintain your balance and stability.

- Bring your hands together at your chest in a prayer position, or extend them overhead like the branches of a tree.

- Hold the pose for 30-60 seconds, focusing on steady breaths and maintaining stability.

- Repeat the exercise on the other leg, aiming for three sets on each side.

Integrating balance and stability exercises into your daily routine is essential for managing knee arthritis and reducing the risk of falls. The five extensively effective exercises mentioned above - single leg stance, heel-to-toe walk, standing leg swings, Tai Chi, and the Tree pose - specifically target balance and stability. You can enhance your balance, coordination, and overall stability by incorporating these exercises into your routine and gradually progressing as your abilities improve. Remember to start slowly, listen to your body, and practice consistently to reap the maximum benefits of these exercises. Improved balance and stability will contribute to a safer and more enjoyable daily life.

Five Minutes Enhancing Flexibility Exercises for Knee Arthritis

Flexibility is crucial in maintaining joint health and mobility, especially for individuals with knee arthritis. Incorporating flexibility exercises into your routine can help improve your range of motion, reduce stiffness, and alleviate knee discomfort. This comprehensive guide will explore five extensively effective flexibility exercises specifically designed to target the muscles and connective tissues around the knees. These exercises can be easily integrated into your daily routine and offer numerous benefits for enhancing flexibility and joint function.

Exercise 19: Quadriceps Stretch

The quadriceps stretch targets the front thigh muscles and help relieve tension in the quadriceps and knee joints. Follow these steps to perform the quadriceps stretch:

- Stand tall and hold onto a sturdy object, such as a wall or chair, for balance.

- Bend your right knee and grasp your right foot or ankle with your right hand.

- Feel a stretch in your front thigh as you slowly pull your foot towards your buttocks.

- Keep your knees close together and maintain an upright posture.

- Release the stretch after 20 to 30 seconds

- Repeat the stretch on the left leg, aiming for three sets on each side.

Exercise 20: Hamstring Stretch

The hamstring stretch targets the muscles at the back of the thigh, promoting flexibility and reducing strain on the knees. Here's how to perform the hamstring stretch:

- Straighten your back while sitting on the edge of a chair with your feet flat on the ground.

- Your right leg should be straight out in front of you, with the heel on the ground.

- Keep your toes pointing upwards and flex your foot.

- Lean forward from your hips, reaching towards your toes while maintaining a slight bend in your knee.

- Observe how your back thigh is being stretched.

- After holding the stretch for 20 to 30 seconds, switch legs.

- Repeat the stretch on the left leg, aiming for three sets on each side.

Exercise 21: Calf Stretch

The calf stretch targets the calf muscles, which play an important role in knee stability and range of motion. Follow these steps to perform the calf stretch:

- Put your hands on the wall at shoulder height while facing the wall.

- Step back with your right foot, keeping both heels flat.

- Keep your right leg straight and slightly bend your left knee.

- Lean forward, allowing your body weight to shift towards the wall.

- Your right calf should feel stretched.

- Sustain the stretch for 20-30 seconds and then switch legs.

- Repeat the stretch on the left leg, aiming for three sets on each side.

Exercise 22: IT Band Stretch

The IT (iliotibial) band stretch targets the connective tissue outside the thigh, which can become tight and contribute to knee discomfort. Here's how to execute the IT band stretch:

- For support, sit next to a solid wall or other object.
- Your right leg should be crossed behind your left.
- Extend your right arm overhead and lean towards the left side, creating a gentle stretch along the right side of your body.
- Feel the stretch along the outer part of your right thigh.
- After 20 to 30 seconds, hold the stretch for the opposite side.
- Repeat the stretch on the left leg, aiming for three sets on each side.

Exercise 23: Seated Knee Hug

The seated knee hug exercise targets the hip flexors and lower back, promoting flexibility and relieving knee tension. Follow these steps to perform the seated knee hug:

- Straighten your back while sitting on the edge of a chair with your feet flat on the ground.
- Lift your right knee towards your chest, using both hands to hug it.
- Keep your back straight, and your shoulders relaxed.
- Feel the stretch in your hip flexors and lower back.
- Sustain the stretch for 20-30 seconds and then switch legs.
- Repeat the stretch on the left leg, aiming for three sets on each side.

Incorporating flexibility exercises into your routine is crucial for individuals with knee arthritis as it helps improve their range of motion, reduce stiffness, and alleviate discomfort. The five extensively effective flexibility exercises mentioned above - quadriceps stretch, hamstring stretch, calf stretch, IT band stretch, and seated knee hug - target the key muscle groups and connective tissues around the knees. By performing these exercises regularly and gradually increasing the intensity and duration, you can enhance your flexibility, promote joint health, and experience greater comfort in daily activities. Remember to listen to your body, start slowly, and adapt the exercises to your comfort level. Improved flexibility will contribute to better knee function and overall well-being.

Cool-Down and Stretching

After completing the 5-minute exercise routine, cooling down and stretching is essential to bring your heart rate and breathing back to normal gradually. Here's how to properly cool down and stretch:

- Perform low-intensity movements such as walking slowly or performing gentle stretching exercises.
- Focus on stretching the major muscle groups, holding each stretch for 20-30 seconds.
- Take deep breaths and allow your body to relax and recover.
- Use this time to reflect on your workout, notice any improvements, and set goals for future sessions.

Lifestyle Tips for Managing Knee Arthritis

Living with knee arthritis requires a multifaceted approach to managing symptoms and maintaining joint health. Along with medical interventions and exercise, healthy lifestyle habits can significantly reduce pain, improved mobility, and overall well-being. This extensive guide will explore six lifestyle tips specifically tailored to managing knee arthritis: weight management, joint protection strategies, healthy diet and nutrition, stress management, adequate rest, and ergonomic modifications. Implementing these strategies into your daily routine can optimize your quality of life and effectively manage knee arthritis.

1. Weight Management:

Maintaining a healthy weight is crucial for individuals with knee arthritis, as excess weight stresses the joints, leading to increased pain and inflammation. Here are some seasoned tips for weight management:

- Consult with a healthcare professional or a registered dietitian to determine an appropriate weight range for your body type.

- Maintain a healthy, balanced diet high in fruits, vegetables, whole grains, lean proteins, and good fats.

- Limit the consumption of processed foods, sugary drinks, and foods high in saturated fats.

- Practice portion control and mindful eating to prevent overeating.

- Engage in regular physical activity, such as low-impact exercises, to aid weight management and strengthen the supporting muscles around the knee joints.

2. **Joint Protection Strategies:** Joint protection strategies can help minimize knee stress and prevent further damage. Consider the following techniques:

- Avoid activities that strain the knees, such as running or jumping.

- Use assistive devices like braces, canes, or walkers to provide additional support and stability.

- Practice proper body mechanics when lifting heavy objects or performing daily tasks, such as bending at the knees and using your leg muscles instead of your back.

- Opt for low-impact exercises like swimming, cycling, or water aerobics that provide cardiovascular benefits without stressing the joints.

- Modify your environment to reduce joint stress by using cushioned mats, ergonomic chairs, or adjustable-height workstations.

3. Healthy Diet and Nutrition:

Maintaining a healthy diet and proper nutrition is vital for managing knee arthritis. Consider the following dietary recommendations:

- Incorporate anti-inflammatory foods into your diet, including fatty fish (such as salmon), nuts, seeds, olive oil, fruits, and vegetables.

- Consume foods rich in omega-3 fatty acids, such as flaxseeds, chia seeds, and walnuts, as they have been shown to reduce inflammation.

- Make sure to consume enough calcium and vitamin D to support the health of your bones. Excellent sources of these nutrients include dairy products, leafy greens, and foods that have been fortified.

- Limit the consumption of foods high in refined sugars, processed grains, and unhealthy fats, as they can promote inflammation.

- Stay hydrated by drinking plenty of water throughout the day to help maintain joint lubrication and overall health.

4. Stress Management:

Chronic pain from knee arthritis can take a toll on mental and emotional well-being. Implementing stress management techniques can help improve overall quality of life. Consider the following strategies:

- Practice relaxation techniques such as deep breathing, meditation, or yoga to reduce stress and promote a sense of calm.

- Engage in activities that bring joy and relaxation, such as hobbies, listening to music, spending time in nature, or engaging in creative outlets.

- Seek support from friends, family, or support groups to share experiences, seek advice, and find emotional support.
- Consider consulting with a mental health professional specializing in chronic pain management to develop effective coping strategies.

5. Adequate Rest:

Getting enough rest is essential for managing knee arthritis as it allows the body to heal and recharge. Follow these tips for better sleep and rest:

- Keep a regular sleep schedule and aim for 7-8 hours of restful sleep each night.
- Create a comfortable sleep environment by investing in a supportive mattress, pillows, and appropriate bedding.
- Practice good sleep hygiene, such as avoiding electronic devices before bed, keeping the bedroom dark and quiet, and establishing a relaxing bedtime routine.
- If knee pain disrupts sleep, use pillows or cushions to elevate the affected leg and reduce discomfort.

6. Ergonomic Modifications:

Making ergonomic modifications in your daily life can significantly reduce knee strain and improve overall comfort. Consider the following adjustments:

- Ensure proper ergonomics by using an adjustable chair, maintaining good posture, and positioning your workstation at the appropriate height.
- Use supportive footwear with cushioned soles and adequate arch support to minimize the impact on the knees during walking or standing.
- Install handrails or grab bars in areas of the home where extra support and stability are needed, such as staircases or bathrooms.
- To minimize joint stress and strain, use assistive devices for daily activities, such as jar openers, reachers, or long-handled tools.

Incorporating these lifestyle tips into your daily routine can significantly improve your ability to manage knee arthritis effectively. Weight management, joint protection strategies, healthy diet and nutrition, stress management, adequate rest, and ergonomic modifications are crucial in minimizing pain, maintaining joint health, and optimizing overall well-being. Remember to consult with healthcare professionals, such as physicians, physical therapists, and dietitians, for personalized advice and guidance. By embracing a holistic approach to knee arthritis management, you can take control of your condition and lead a fulfilling and active life.

Conclusion

This comprehensive guide has explored various aspects of managing knee arthritis, providing valuable insights and practical advice for seniors over 50. From understanding the nature of knee arthritis to exploring treatment options and lifestyle strategies, this book aims to empower individuals to take control of their condition and enhance their quality of life.

We began by delving into the definition of knee arthritis and its causes, shedding light on the factors contributing to its development. We then examined the symptoms and diagnosis process, emphasizing the importance of early detection and seeking medical attention.

We focused on treatment options and introduced the concept of a pain-free exercise routine specifically designed for seniors. This 5-minute exercise routine, with its low-impact aerobic exercises, range of motion exercises, strengthening exercises, balance and stability exercises, and flexibility exercises, provides a practical and manageable solution for managing knee arthritis.

Understanding the significance of lifestyle factors in managing knee arthritis, we discussed weight management, joint protection strategies, healthy diet and nutrition, stress management, adequate rest, and ergonomic modifications. By integrating these lifestyle tips into daily routines, individuals can maximize the benefits of exercise and optimize their overall well-being.

knee arthritis may present challenges, but with knowledge, commitment, and the right approach, it is possible to live a fulfilling and pain-free life. By utilizing the information and strategies shared in this book, seniors over 50 can regain control of their knee health, alleviate discomfort, and enjoy an active and vibrant lifestyle. Remember, taking small steps each day can lead to significant improvements. With perseverance, you can overcome the limitations of knee arthritis and embrace a future filled with vitality and freedom.

Book's Picture Links

https://www.pexels.com/photo/elderly-couple-walking-by-the-bay-5637806/

https://www.pexels.com/photo/close-up-shot-of-a-wounded-knee-7298467/

https://images.pexels.com/photos/8638040/pexels-photo-8638040.jpeg?auto=compress&cs=tinysrgb&w=1260&h=750&dpr=1

BONUS

<u>EXERCISE TRACKER</u>

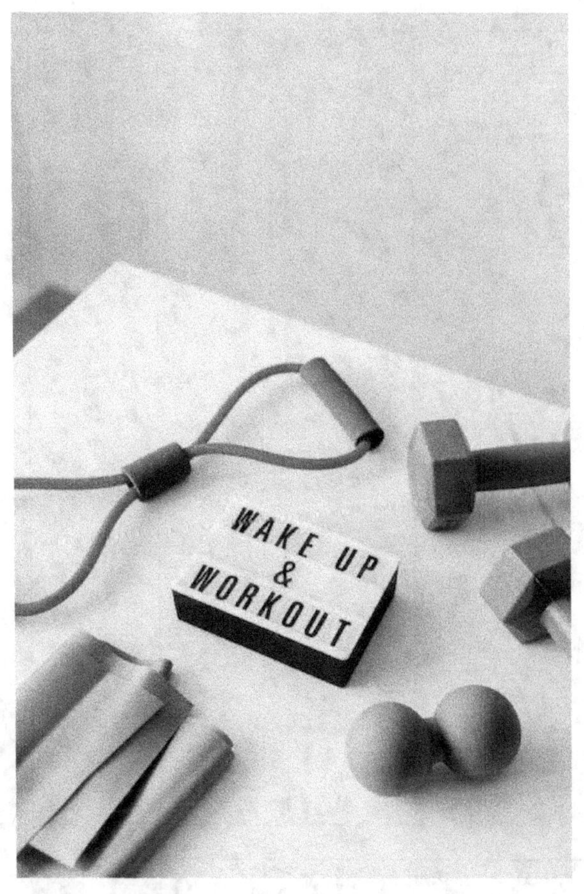

WORKOUT LOG

NAME:
GOALS:
DATE:
STATS:
WEIGHT:

EXERCISE:	SETS	REPS	WEIGHT	REST	SETS	REPS	WEIGHT	REST	SETS	REPS	WEIGHT	REST	SETS	REPS	WEIGHT	REST

CARDIO:	TIME	DIST.	INT.	PACE	TIME	DIST.	INT.	PACE	TIME	DIST.	INT.	PACE	TIME	DIST.	INT.	PACE

WORKOUT LOG

NAME:
GOALS:
DATE:
STATS:
WEIGHT:

EXERCISE:	SETS	REPS	WEIGHT	REST	SETS	REPS	WEIGHT	REST	SETS	REPS	WEIGHT	REST	SETS	REPS	WEIGHT	REST

CARDIO:	TIME	DIST.	INT.	PACE	TIME	DIST.	INT.	PACE	TIME	DIST.	INT.	PACE	TIME	DIST.	INT.	PACE

WORKOUT LOG

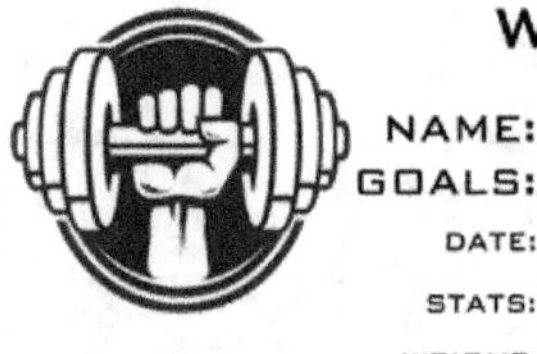

NAME:

GOALS:

DATE:

STATS:

WEIGHT:

EXERCISE:	SETS	REPS	WEIGHT	REST	SETS	REPS	WEIGHT	REST	SETS	REPS	WEIGHT	REST	SETS	REPS	WEIGHT	REST

CARDIO:	TIME	DIST.	INT.	PACE	TIME	DIST.	INT.	PACE	TIME	DIST.	INT.	PACE	TIME	DIST.	INT.	PACE

WORKOUT LOG

NAME:
GOALS:
DATE:
STATS:
WEIGHT:

EXERCISE:	SETS	REPS	WEIGHT	REST	SETS	REPS	WEIGHT	REST	SETS	REPS	WEIGHT	REST	SETS	REPS	WEIGHT	REST

CARDIO:	TIME	DIST.	INT.	PACE	TIME	DIST.	INT.	PACE	TIME	DIST.	INT.	PACE	TIME	DIST.	INT.	PACE

WORKOUT LOG

NAME:

GOALS:

DATE:

STATS:

WEIGHT:

EXERCISE:	SETS	REPS	WEIGHT	REST	SETS	REPS	WEIGHT	REST	SETS	REPS	WEIGHT	REST	SETS	REPS	WEIGHT	REST

CARDIO:	TIME	DIST.	INT.	PACE	TIME	DIST.	INT.	PACE	TIME	DIST.	INT.	PACE	TIME	DIST.	INT.	PACE

WORKOUT LOG

NAME:
GOALS:
DATE:
STATS:
WEIGHT:

EXERCISE:	SETS	REPS	WEIGHT	REST	SETS	REPS	WEIGHT	REST	SETS	REPS	WEIGHT	REST	SETS	REPS	WEIGHT	REST

CARDIO:	TIME	DIST.	INT.	PACE	TIME	DIST.	INT.	PACE	TIME	DIST.	INT.	PACE	TIME	DIST.	INT.	PACE

WORKOUT LOG

NAME: _______________________________

GOALS: _______________________________

DATE:

STATS:

WEIGHT:

EXERCISE:	SETS	REPS	WEIGHT	REST	SETS	REPS	WEIGHT	REST	SETS	REPS	WEIGHT	REST	SETS	REPS	WEIGHT	REST

CARDIO:	TIME	DIST.	INT.	PACE	TIME	DIST.	INT.	PACE	TIME	DIST.	INT.	PACE	TIME	DIST.	INT.	PACE

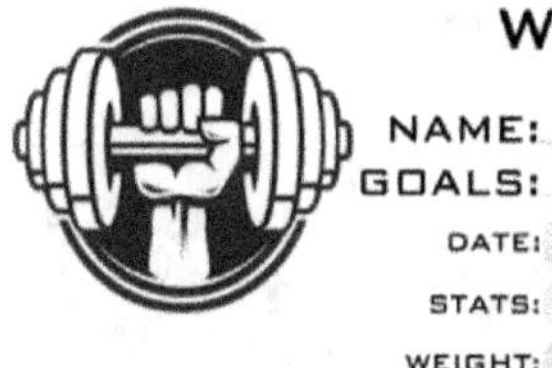

WORKOUT LOG

NAME:

GOALS:

DATE:

STATS:

WEIGHT:

EXERCISE:	SETS	REPS	WEIGHT	REST	SETS	REPS	WEIGHT	REST	SETS	REPS	WEIGHT	REST	SETS	REPS	WEIGHT	REST

CARDIO:	TIME	DIST.	INT.	PACE	TIME	DIST.	INT.	PACE	TIME	DIST.	INT.	PACE	TIME	DIST.	INT.	PACE

WORKOUT LOG

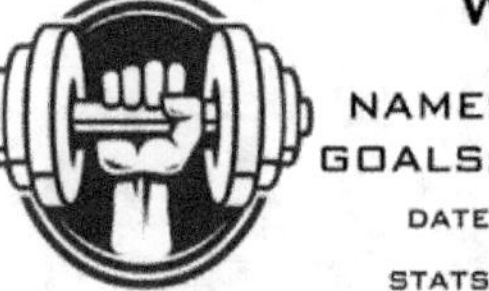

NAME:

GOALS:

DATE:

STATS:

WEIGHT:

EXERCISE:	SETS	REPS	WEIGHT	REST	SETS	REPS	WEIGHT	REST	SETS	REPS	WEIGHT	REST	SETS	REPS	WEIGHT	REST

CARDIO:	TIME	DIST.	INT.	PACE	TIME	DIST.	INT.	PACE	TIME	DIST.	INT.	PACE	TIME	DIST.	INT.	PACE

WORKOUT LOG

NAME:

GOALS:

DATE:

STATS:

WEIGHT:

EXERCISE:	SETS	REPS	WEIGHT	REST	SETS	REPS	WEIGHT	REST	SETS	REPS	WEIGHT	REST	SETS	REPS	WEIGHT	REST

CARDIO:	TIME	DIST.	INT.	PACE	TIME	DIST.	INT.	PACE	TIME	DIST.	INT.	PACE	TIME	DIST.	INT.	PACE